TIER FIT

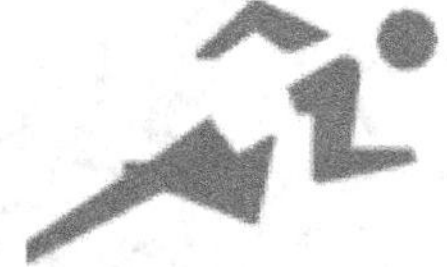

NAME:

DATE:

TIME START:

TIME END:

WARM-UP	TIME	NOTES

STRETCH:	TIME	NOTES

EXERCISE:	SET 1		SET 2		SET 3		SET 4	
	REPS	WEIGHT	REPS	WEIGHT	REPS	WEIGHT	REPS	WEIGHT

CARDIO:	TIME	DISTANCE	PACE	HR

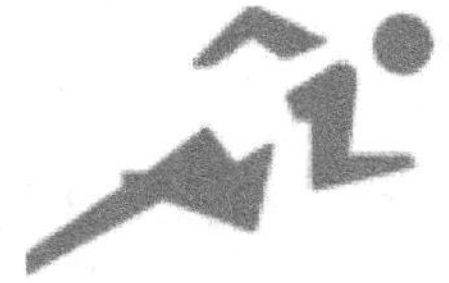

NAME:

DATE:

TIME START:

TIME END:

WARM-UP	TIME	NOTES

STRETCH:	TIME	NOTES

EXERCISE:	SET 1		SET 2		SET 3		SET 4	
	REPS	WEIGHT	REPS	WEIGHT	REPS	WEIGHT	REPS	WEIGHT

CARDIO:	TIME	DISTANCE	PACE	HR

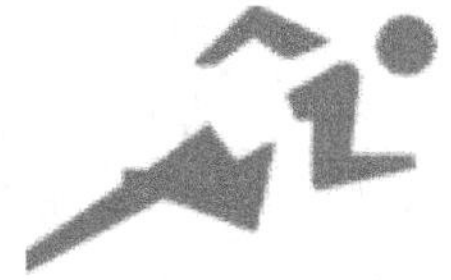

NAME:

DATE:

TIME START:

TIME END:

WARM-UP	TIME	NOTES

STRETCH:	TIME	NOTES

EXERCISE:	SET 1		SET 2		SET 3		SET 4	
	REPS	WEIGHT	REPS	WEIGHT	REPS	WEIGHT	REPS	WEIGHT

CARDIO:	TIME	DISTANCE	PACE	HR

NAME:

DATE:

TIME START:

TIME END:

WARM-UP	TIME	NOTES

STRETCH:	TIME	NOTES

EXERCISE:	SET 1		SET 2		SET 3		SET 4	
	REPS	WEIGHT	REPS	WEIGHT	REPS	WEIGHT	REPS	WEIGHT

CARDIO:	TIME	DISTANCE	PACE	HR

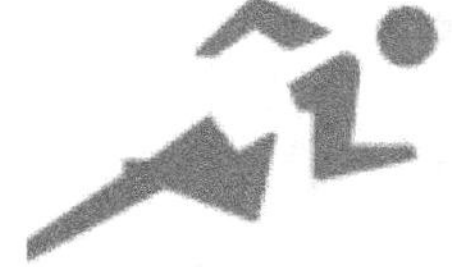

NAME:

DATE:

TIME START:

TIME END:

WARM-UP	TIME	NOTES

STRETCH:	TIME	NOTES

EXERCISE:	SET 1		SET 2		SET 3		SET 4	
	REPS	WEIGHT	REPS	WEIGHT	REPS	WEIGHT	REPS	WEIGHT

CARDIO:	TIME	DISTANCE	PACE	HR

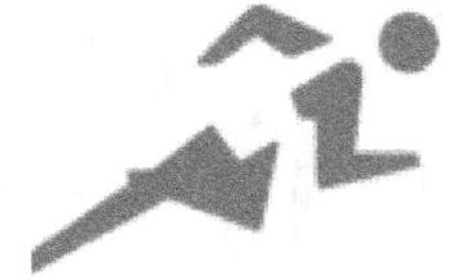

NAME:

DATE:

TIME START:

TIME END:

WARM-UP	TIME	NOTES

STRETCH:	TIME	NOTES

EXERCISE:	SET 1		SET 2		SET 3		SET 4	
	REPS	WEIGHT	REPS	WEIGHT	REPS	WEIGHT	REPS	WEIGHT

CARDIO:	TIME	DISTANCE	PACE	HR

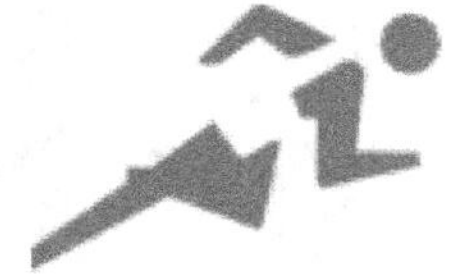

NAME:

DATE:

TIME START:

TIME END:

WARM-UP	TIME	NOTES

STRETCH:	TIME	NOTES

EXERCISE:	SET 1		SET 2		SET 3		SET 4	
	REPS	WEIGHT	REPS	WEIGHT	REPS	WEIGHT	REPS	WEIGHT

CARDIO:	TIME	DISTANCE	PACE	HR

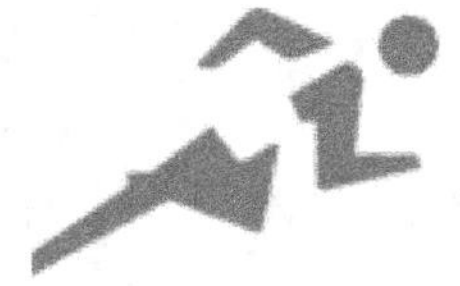

NAME:

DATE:

TIME START:

TIME END:

WARM-UP	TIME	NOTES

STRETCH:	TIME	NOTES

EXERCISE:	SET 1		SET 2		SET 3		SET 4	
	REPS	WEIGHT	REPS	WEIGHT	REPS	WEIGHT	REPS	WEIGHT

CARDIO:	TIME	DISTANCE	PACE	HR

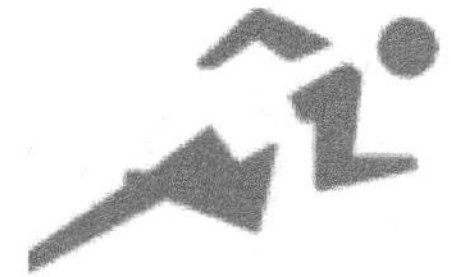

NAME: ________________________

DATE: ________________________

TIME START: ________________________

TIME END: ________________________

WARM-UP	TIME	NOTES

STRETCH:	TIME	NOTES

EXERCISE:	SET 1		SET 2		SET 3		SET 4	
	REPS	WEIGHT	REPS	WEIGHT	REPS	WEIGHT	REPS	WEIGHT

CARDIO:	TIME	DISTANCE	PACE	HR

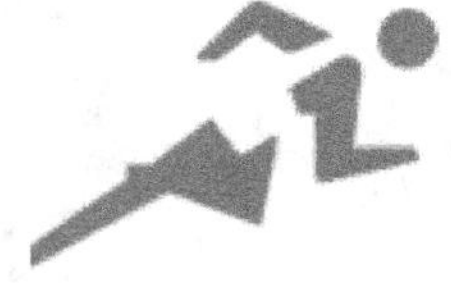

NAME:

DATE:

TIME START:

TIME END:

WARM-UP	TIME	NOTES

STRETCH:	TIME	NOTES

EXERCISE:	SET 1		SET 2		SET 3		SET 4	
	REPS	WEIGHT	REPS	WEIGHT	REPS	WEIGHT	REPS	WEIGHT

CARDIO:	TIME	DISTANCE	PACE	HR

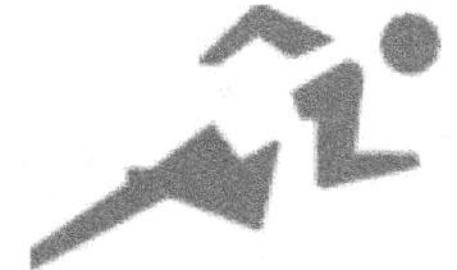

NAME:

DATE:

TIME START:

TIME END:

WARM-UP	TIME	NOTES

STRETCH:	TIME	NOTES

EXERCISE:	SET 1		SET 2		SET 3		SET 4	
	REPS	WEIGHT	REPS	WEIGHT	REPS	WEIGHT	REPS	WEIGHT

CARDIO:	TIME	DISTANCE	PACE	HR

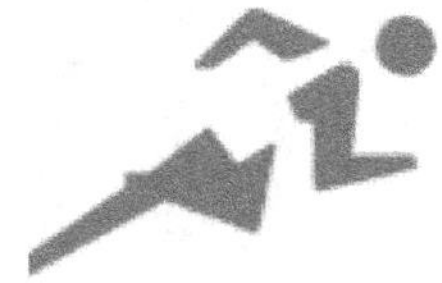

NAME:

DATE:

TIME START:

TIME END:

WARM-UP	TIME	NOTES

STRETCH:	TIME	NOTES

EXERCISE:	SET 1		SET 2		SET 3		SET 4	
	REPS	WEIGHT	REPS	WEIGHT	REPS	WEIGHT	REPS	WEIGHT

CARDIO:	TIME	DISTANCE	PACE	HR

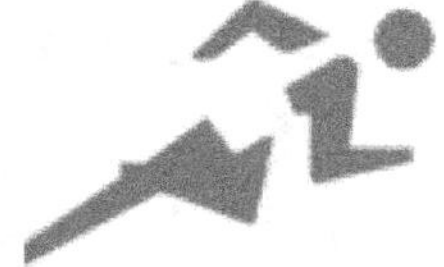

NAME:

DATE:

TIME START:

TIME END:

WARM-UP	TIME	NOTES

STRETCH:	TIME	NOTES

EXERCISE:	SET 1		SET 2		SET 3		SET 4	
	REPS	WEIGHT	REPS	WEIGHT	REPS	WEIGHT	REPS	WEIGHT

CARDIO:	TIME	DISTANCE	PACE	HR

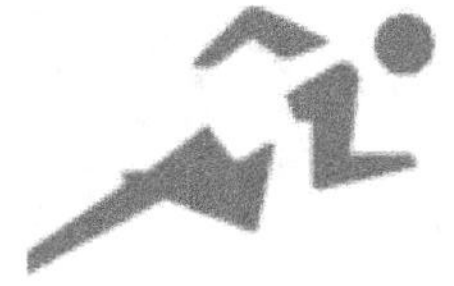

NAME:

DATE:

TIME START:

TIME END:

WARM-UP	TIME	NOTES

STRETCH:	TIME	NOTES

EXERCISE:	SET 1		SET 2		SET 3		SET 4	
	REPS	WEIGHT	REPS	WEIGHT	REPS	WEIGHT	REPS	WEIGHT

CARDIO:	TIME	DISTANCE	PACE	HR

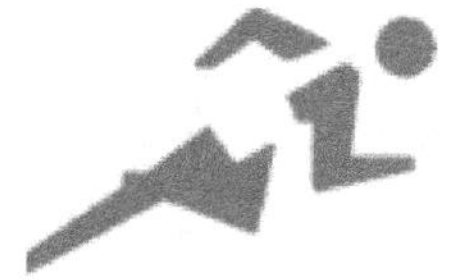

NAME:	
DATE:	
TIME START:	
TIME END:	

WARM-UP	TIME	NOTES

STRETCH:	TIME	NOTES

EXERCISE:	SET 1		SET 2		SET 3		SET 4	
	REPS	WEIGHT	REPS	WEIGHT	REPS	WEIGHT	REPS	WEIGHT

CARDIO:	TIME	DISTANCE	PACE	HR

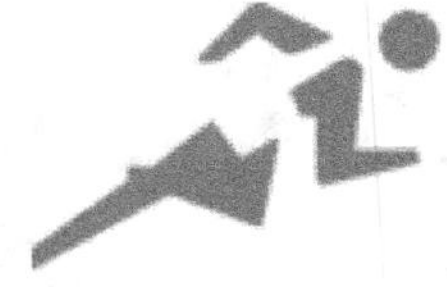

NAME:

DATE:

TIME START:

TIME END:

WARM-UP	TIME	NOTES

STRETCH:	TIME	NOTES

EXERCISE:	SET 1		SET 2		SET 3		SET 4	
	REPS	WEIGHT	REPS	WEIGHT	REPS	WEIGHT	REPS	WEIGHT

CARDIO:	TIME	DISTANCE	PACE	HR

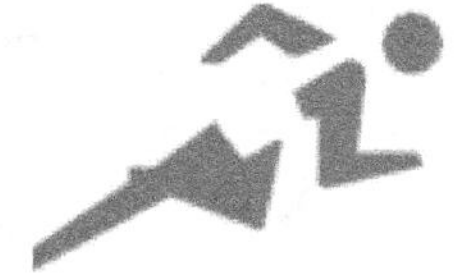

NAME:

DATE:

TIME START:

TIME END:

WARM-UP	TIME	NOTES

STRETCH:	TIME	NOTES

EXERCISE:	SET 1		SET 2		SET 3		SET 4	
	REPS	WEIGHT	REPS	WEIGHT	REPS	WEIGHT	REPS	WEIGHT

CARDIO:	TIME	DISTANCE	PACE	HR

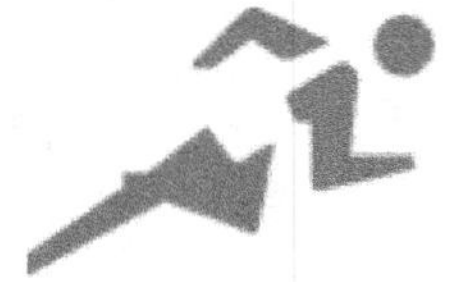

NAME:

DATE:

TIME START:

TIME END:

WARM-UP	TIME	NOTES

STRETCH:	TIME	NOTES

EXERCISE:	SET 1		SET 2		SET 3		SET 4	
	REPS	WEIGHT	REPS	WEIGHT	REPS	WEIGHT	REPS	WEIGHT

CARDIO:	TIME	DISTANCE	PACE	HR

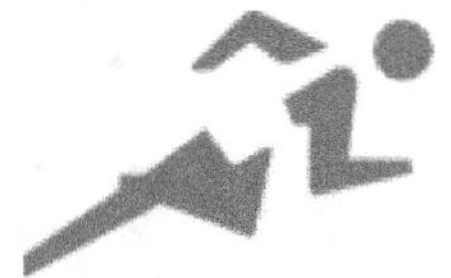

NAME:

DATE:

TIME START:

TIME END:

WARM-UP	TIME	NOTES

STRETCH:	TIME	NOTES

EXERCISE:	SET 1		SET 2		SET 3		SET 4	
	REPS	WEIGHT	REPS	WEIGHT	REPS	WEIGHT	REPS	WEIGHT

CARDIO:	TIME	DISTANCE	PACE	HR

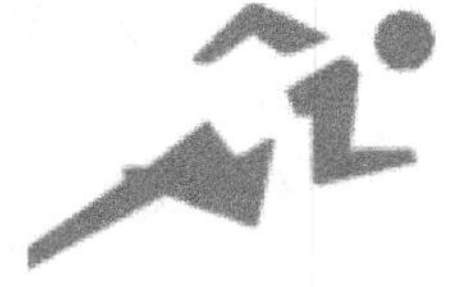

NAME:
DATE:
TIME START:
TIME END:

WARM-UP	TIME	NOTES

STRETCH:	TIME	NOTES

EXERCISE:	SET 1		SET 2		SET 3		SET 4	
	REPS	WEIGHT	REPS	WEIGHT	REPS	WEIGHT	REPS	WEIGHT

CARDIO:	TIME	DISTANCE	PACE	HR

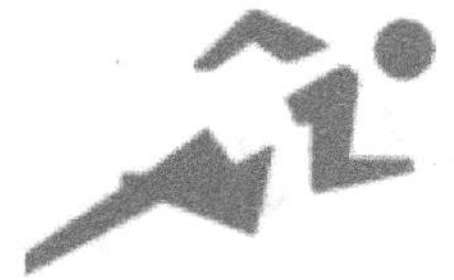

NAME:

DATE:

TIME START:

TIME END:

WARM-UP	TIME	NOTES

STRETCH:	TIME	NOTES

EXERCISE:	SET 1		SET 2		SET 3		SET 4	
	REPS	WEIGHT	REPS	WEIGHT	REPS	WEIGHT	REPS	WEIGHT

CARDIO:	TIME	DISTANCE	PACE	HR

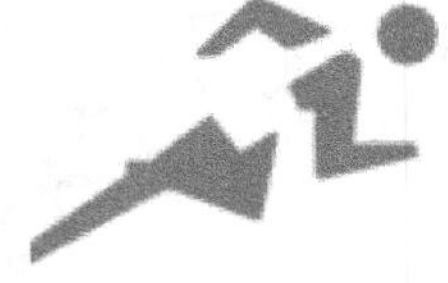

NAME: _______________

DATE: _______________

TIME START: _______________

TIME END: _______________

WARM-UP	TIME	NOTES

STRETCH:	TIME	NOTES

EXERCISE:	SET 1		SET 2		SET 3		SET 4	
	REPS	WEIGHT	REPS	WEIGHT	REPS	WEIGHT	REPS	WEIGHT

CARDIO:	TIME	DISTANCE	PACE	HR

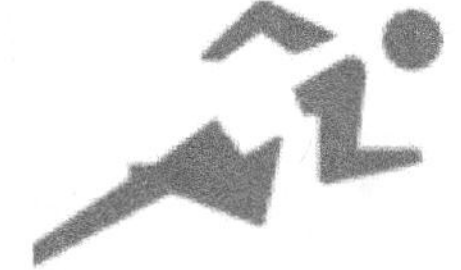

NAME:

DATE:

TIME START:

TIME END:

WARM-UP	TIME	NOTES

STRETCH:	TIME	NOTES

EXERCISE:	SET 1		SET 2		SET 3		SET 4	
	REPS	WEIGHT	REPS	WEIGHT	REPS	WEIGHT	REPS	WEIGHT

CARDIO:	TIME	DISTANCE	PACE	HR

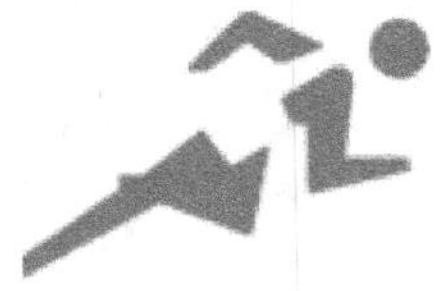

NAME:

DATE:

TIME START:

TIME END:

WARM-UP	TIME	NOTES

STRETCH:	TIME	NOTES

EXERCISE:	SET 1		SET 2		SET 3		SET 4	
	REPS	WEIGHT	REPS	WEIGHT	REPS	WEIGHT	REPS	WEIGHT

CARDIO:	TIME	DISTANCE	PACE	HR

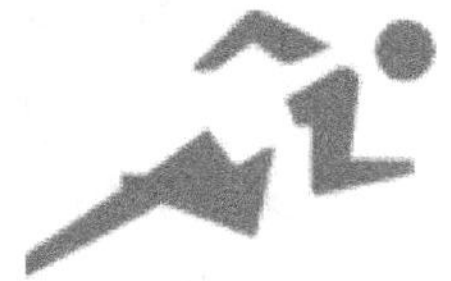

NAME:

DATE:

TIME START:

TIME END:

WARM-UP	TIME	NOTES

STRETCH:	TIME	NOTES

EXERCISE:	SET 1		SET 2		SET 3		SET 4	
	REPS	WEIGHT	REPS	WEIGHT	REPS	WEIGHT	REPS	WEIGHT

CARDIO:	TIME	DISTANCE	PACE	HR

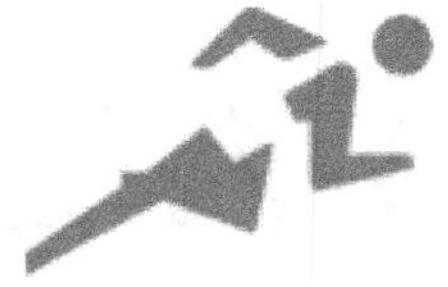

NAME:

DATE:

TIME START:

TIME END:

WARM-UP	TIME	NOTES

STRETCH:	TIME	NOTES

EXERCISE:	SET 1		SET 2		SET 3		SET 4	
	REPS	WEIGHT	REPS	WEIGHT	REPS	WEIGHT	REPS	WEIGHT

CARDIO:	TIME	DISTANCE	PACE	HR

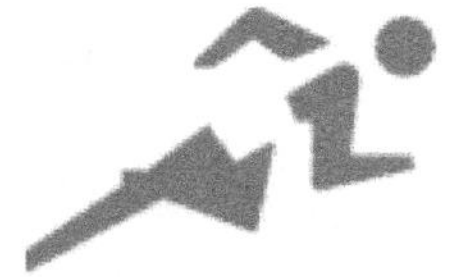

NAME:

DATE:

TIME START:

TIME END:

WARM-UP	TIME	NOTES

STRETCH:	TIME	NOTES

EXERCISE:	SET 1		SET 2		SET 3		SET 4	
	REPS	WEIGHT	REPS	WEIGHT	REPS	WEIGHT	REPS	WEIGHT

CARDIO:	TIME	DISTANCE	PACE	HR

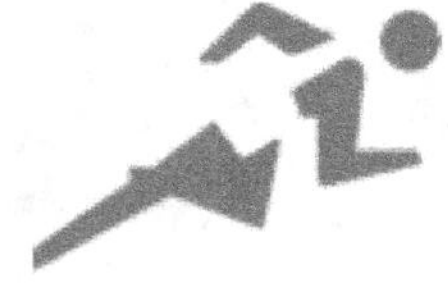

NAME:

DATE:

TIME START:

TIME END:

WARM-UP	TIME	NOTES

STRETCH:	TIME	NOTES

EXERCISE:	SET 1		SET 2		SET 3		SET 4	
	REPS	WEIGHT	REPS	WEIGHT	REPS	WEIGHT	REPS	WEIGHT

CARDIO:	TIME	DISTANCE	PACE	HR

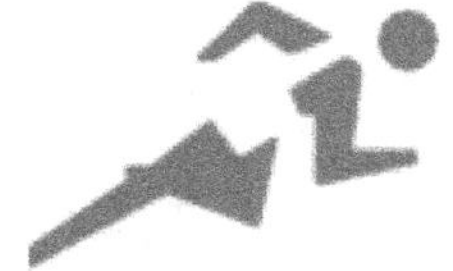

NAME:

DATE:

TIME START:

TIME END:

WARM-UP	TIME	NOTES

STRETCH:	TIME	NOTES

EXERCISE:	SET 1		SET 2		SET 3		SET 4	
	REPS	WEIGHT	REPS	WEIGHT	REPS	WEIGHT	REPS	WEIGHT

CARDIO:	TIME	DISTANCE	PACE	HR

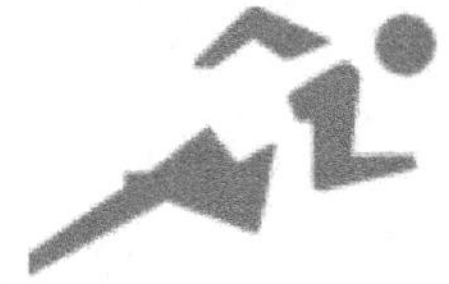

NAME:

DATE:

TIME START:

TIME END:

WARM-UP	TIME	NOTES

STRETCH:	TIME	NOTES

EXERCISE:	SET 1		SET 2		SET 3		SET 4	
	REPS	WEIGHT	REPS	WEIGHT	REPS	WEIGHT	REPS	WEIGHT

CARDIO:	TIME	DISTANCE	PACE	HR

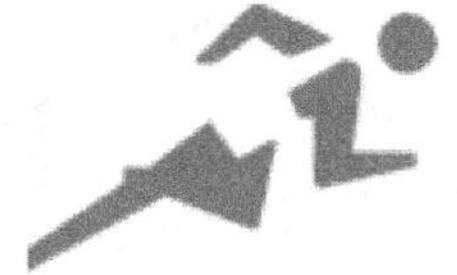

NAME:

DATE:

TIME START:

TIME END:

WARM-UP	TIME	NOTES

STRETCH:	TIME	NOTES

EXERCISE:	SET 1		SET 2		SET 3		SET 4	
	REPS	WEIGHT	REPS	WEIGHT	REPS	WEIGHT	REPS	WEIGHT

CARDIO:	TIME	DISTANCE	PACE	HR

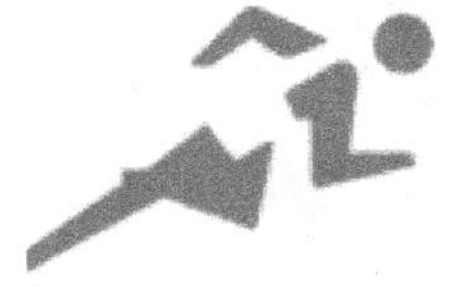

NAME:

DATE:

TIME START:

TIME END:

WARM-UP	TIME	NOTES

STRETCH:	TIME	NOTES

EXERCISE:	SET 1		SET 2		SET 3		SET 4	
	REPS	WEIGHT	REPS	WEIGHT	REPS	WEIGHT	REPS	WEIGHT

CARDIO:	TIME	DISTANCE	PACE	HR

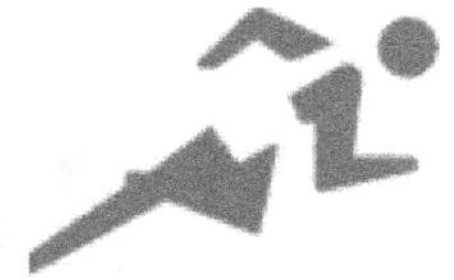

NAME:

DATE:

TIME START:

TIME END:

WARM-UP	TIME	NOTES

STRETCH:	TIME	NOTES

EXERCISE:	SET 1		SET 2		SET 3		SET 4	
	REPS	WEIGHT	REPS	WEIGHT	REPS	WEIGHT	REPS	WEIGHT

CARDIO:	TIME	DISTANCE	PACE	HR

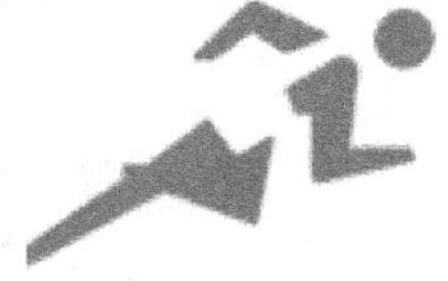

WARM-UP	TIME	NOTES

STRETCH:	TIME	NOTES

EXERCISE:	SET 1		SET 2		SET 3		SET 4	
	REPS	WEIGHT	REPS	WEIGHT	REPS	WEIGHT	REPS	WEIGHT

CARDIO:	TIME	DISTANCE	PACE	HR

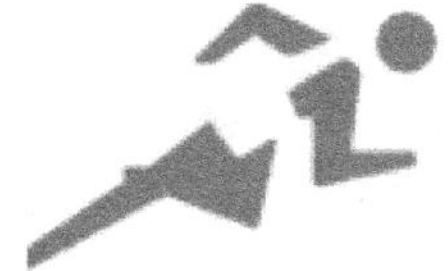

NAME:

DATE:

TIME START:

TIME END:

WARM-UP	TIME	NOTES

STRETCH:	TIME	NOTES

EXERCISE:	SET 1		SET 2		SET 3		SET 4	
	REPS	WEIGHT	REPS	WEIGHT	REPS	WEIGHT	REPS	WEIGHT

CARDIO:	TIME	DISTANCE	PACE	HR

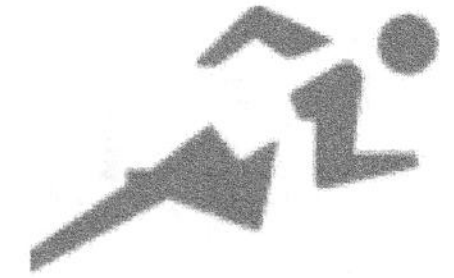

NAME: ___________

DATE: ___________

TIME START: ___________

TIME END: ___________

WARM-UP	TIME	NOTES

STRETCH:	TIME	NOTES

EXERCISE:	SET 1		SET 2		SET 3		SET 4	
	REPS	WEIGHT	REPS	WEIGHT	REPS	WEIGHT	REPS	WEIGHT

CARDIO:	TIME	DISTANCE	PACE	HR

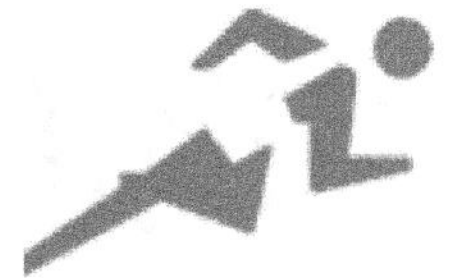

NAME:

DATE:

TIME START:

TIME END:

WARM-UP	TIME	NOTES

STRETCH:	TIME	NOTES

EXERCISE:	SET 1		SET 2		SET 3		SET 4	
	REPS	WEIGHT	REPS	WEIGHT	REPS	WEIGHT	REPS	WEIGHT

CARDIO:	TIME	DISTANCE	PACE	HR

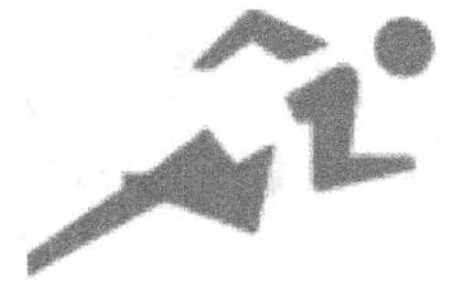

NAME:

DATE:

TIME START:

TIME END:

WARM-UP	TIME	NOTES

STRETCH:	TIME	NOTES

EXERCISE:	SET 1		SET 2		SET 3		SET 4	
	REPS	WEIGHT	REPS	WEIGHT	REPS	WEIGHT	REPS	WEIGHT

CARDIO:	TIME	DISTANCE	PACE	HR

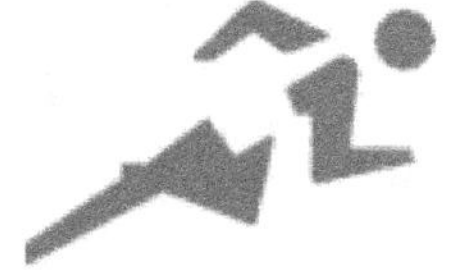

NAME:

DATE:

TIME START:

TIME END:

WARM-UP	TIME	NOTES

STRETCH:	TIME	NOTES

EXERCISE:	SET 1		SET 2		SET 3		SET 4	
	REPS	WEIGHT	REPS	WEIGHT	REPS	WEIGHT	REPS	WEIGHT

CARDIO:	TIME	DISTANCE	PACE	HR

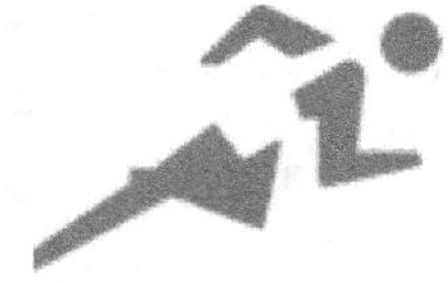

NAME: _______________

DATE: _______________

TIME START: _______________

TIME END: _______________

WARM-UP	TIME	NOTES

STRETCH:	TIME	NOTES

EXERCISE:	SET 1		SET 2		SET 3		SET 4	
	REPS	WEIGHT	REPS	WEIGHT	REPS	WEIGHT	REPS	WEIGHT

CARDIO:	TIME	DISTANCE	PACE	HR

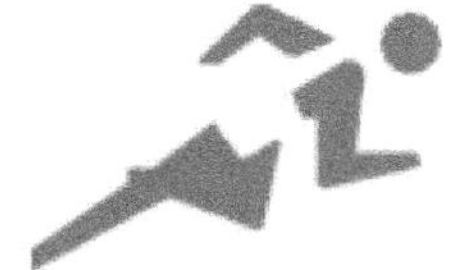

NAME:

DATE:

TIME START:

TIME END:

WARM-UP	TIME	NOTES

STRETCH:	TIME	NOTES

EXERCISE:	SET 1		SET 2		SET 3		SET 4	
	REPS	WEIGHT	REPS	WEIGHT	REPS	WEIGHT	REPS	WEIGHT

CARDIO:	TIME	DISTANCE	PACE	HR

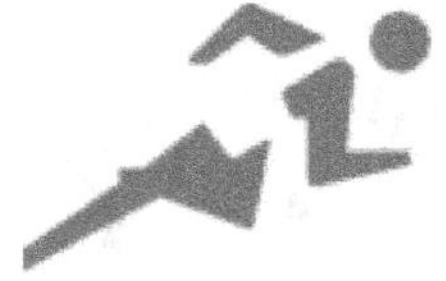

NAME:

DATE:

TIME START:

TIME END:

WARM-UP	TIME	NOTES

STRETCH:	TIME	NOTES

EXERCISE:	SET 1		SET 2		SET 3		SET 4	
	REPS	WEIGHT	REPS	WEIGHT	REPS	WEIGHT	REPS	WEIGHT

CARDIO:	TIME	DISTANCE	PACE	HR

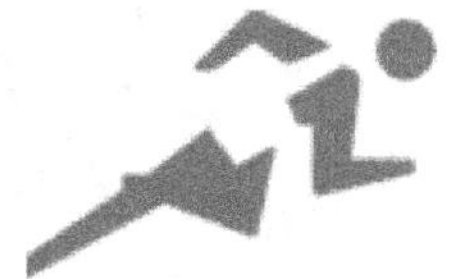

NAME:

DATE:

TIME START:

TIME END:

WARM-UP	TIME	NOTES

STRETCH:	TIME	NOTES

EXERCISE:	SET 1		SET 2		SET 3		SET 4	
	REPS	WEIGHT	REPS	WEIGHT	REPS	WEIGHT	REPS	WEIGHT

CARDIO:	TIME	DISTANCE	PACE	HR

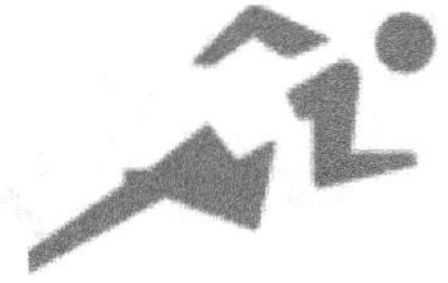

WARM-UP	TIME	NOTES

STRETCH:	TIME	NOTES

EXERCISE:	SET 1		SET 2		SET 3		SET 4	
	REPS	WEIGHT	REPS	WEIGHT	REPS	WEIGHT	REPS	WEIGHT

CARDIO:	TIME	DISTANCE	PACE	HR

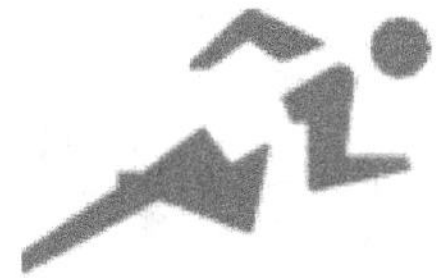

NAME:

DATE:

TIME START:

TIME END:

WARM-UP	TIME	NOTES

STRETCH:	TIME	NOTES

EXERCISE:	SET 1		SET 2		SET 3		SET 4	
	REPS	WEIGHT	REPS	WEIGHT	REPS	WEIGHT	REPS	WEIGHT

CARDIO:	TIME	DISTANCE	PACE	HR

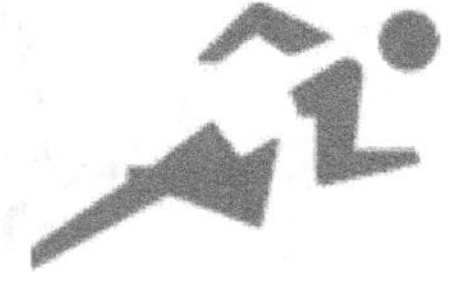

NAME:

DATE:

TIME START:

TIME END:

WARM-UP	TIME	NOTES

STRETCH:	TIME	NOTES

EXERCISE:	SET 1		SET 2		SET 3		SET 4	
	REPS	WEIGHT	REPS	WEIGHT	REPS	WEIGHT	REPS	WEIGHT

CARDIO:	TIME	DISTANCE	PACE	HR

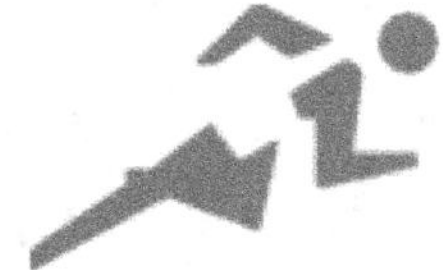

NAME:

DATE:

TIME START:

TIME END:

WARM-UP	TIME	NOTES

STRETCH:	TIME	NOTES

EXERCISE:	SET 1		SET 2		SET 3		SET 4	
	REPS	WEIGHT	REPS	WEIGHT	REPS	WEIGHT	REPS	WEIGHT

CARDIO:	TIME	DISTANCE	PACE	HR

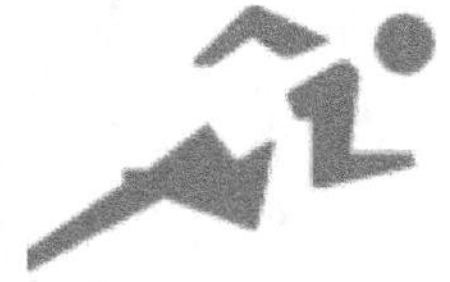

NAME:

DATE:

TIME START:

TIME END:

WARM-UP	TIME	NOTES

STRETCH:	TIME	NOTES

EXERCISE:	SET 1		SET 2		SET 3		SET 4	
	REPS	WEIGHT	REPS	WEIGHT	REPS	WEIGHT	REPS	WEIGHT

CARDIO:	TIME	DISTANCE	PACE	HR

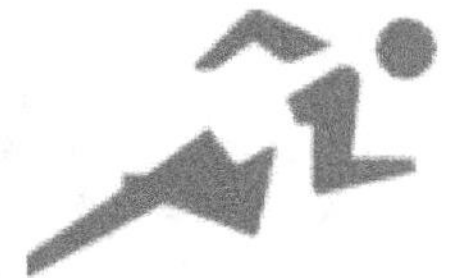

NAME:

DATE:

TIME START:

TIME END:

WARM-UP	TIME	NOTES

STRETCH:	TIME	NOTES

EXERCISE:	SET 1		SET 2		SET 3		SET 4	
	REPS	WEIGHT	REPS	WEIGHT	REPS	WEIGHT	REPS	WEIGHT

CARDIO:	TIME	DISTANCE	PACE	HR

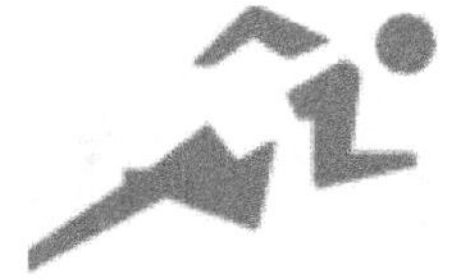

NAME:

DATE:

TIME START:

TIME END:

WARM-UP	TIME	NOTES

STRETCH:	TIME	NOTES

EXERCISE:	SET 1		SET 2		SET 3		SET 4	
	REPS	WEIGHT	REPS	WEIGHT	REPS	WEIGHT	REPS	WEIGHT

CARDIO:	TIME	DISTANCE	PACE	HR

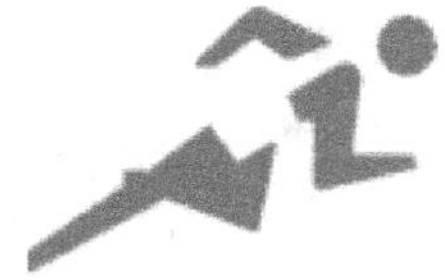

NAME: ______________________

DATE: ______________________

TIME START: ________________

TIME END: __________________

WARM-UP	TIME	NOTES

STRETCH:	TIME	NOTES

EXERCISE:	SET 1		SET 2		SET 3		SET 4	
	REPS	WEIGHT	REPS	WEIGHT	REPS	WEIGHT	REPS	WEIGHT

CARDIO:	TIME	DISTANCE	PACE	HR

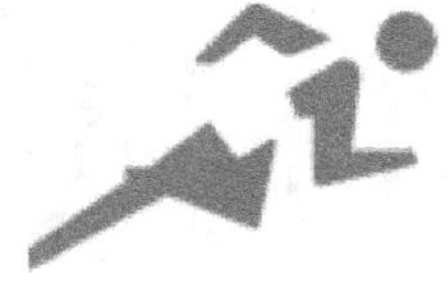

NAME:

DATE:

TIME START:

TIME END:

WARM-UP	TIME	NOTES

STRETCH:	TIME	NOTES

EXERCISE:	SET 1		SET 2		SET 3		SET 4	
	REPS	WEIGHT	REPS	WEIGHT	REPS	WEIGHT	REPS	WEIGHT

CARDIO:	TIME	DISTANCE	PACE	HR

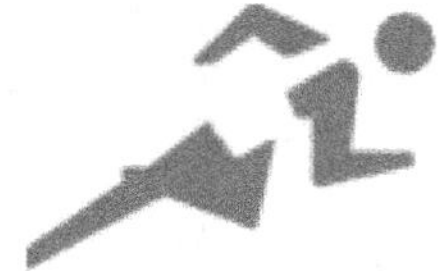

NAME:

DATE:

TIME START:

TIME END:

WARM-UP	TIME	NOTES

STRETCH:	TIME	NOTES

EXERCISE:	SET 1		SET 2		SET 3		SET 4	
	REPS	WEIGHT	REPS	WEIGHT	REPS	WEIGHT	REPS	WEIGHT

CARDIO:	TIME	DISTANCE	PACE	HR

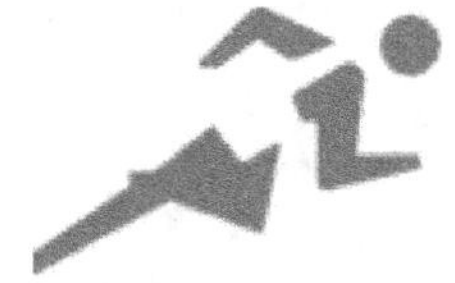

NAME:
DATE:
TIME START:
TIME END:

WARM-UP	TIME	NOTES

STRETCH:	TIME	NOTES

EXERCISE:	SET 1		SET 2		SET 3		SET 4	
	REPS	WEIGHT	REPS	WEIGHT	REPS	WEIGHT	REPS	WEIGHT

CARDIO:	TIME	DISTANCE	PACE	HR

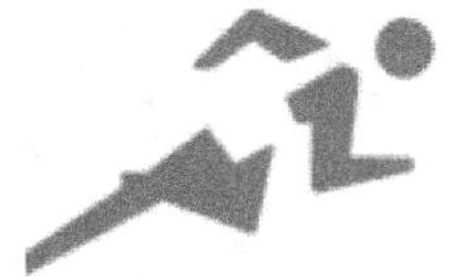

NAME:

DATE:

TIME START:

TIME END:

WARM-UP	TIME	NOTES

STRETCH:	TIME	NOTES

EXERCISE:	SET 1		SET 2		SET 3		SET 4	
	REPS	WEIGHT	REPS	WEIGHT	REPS	WEIGHT	REPS	WEIGHT

CARDIO:	TIME	DISTANCE	PACE	HR

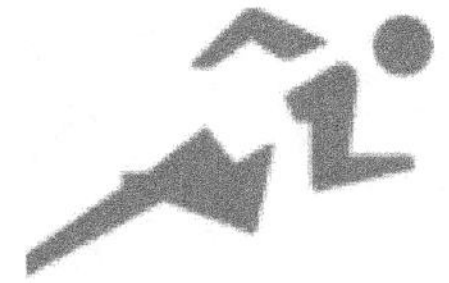

NAME:

DATE:

TIME START:

TIME END:

WARM-UP	TIME	NOTES

STRETCH:	TIME	NOTES

EXERCISE:	SET 1		SET 2		SET 3		SET 4	
	REPS	WEIGHT	REPS	WEIGHT	REPS	WEIGHT	REPS	WEIGHT

CARDIO:	TIME	DISTANCE	PACE	HR

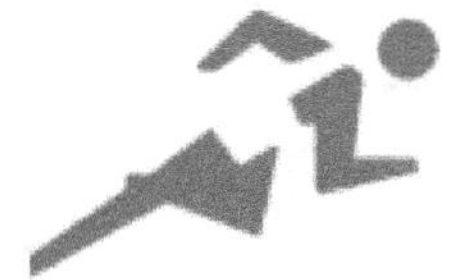

NAME:

DATE:

TIME START:

TIME END:

WARM-UP	TIME	NOTES

STRETCH:	TIME	NOTES

EXERCISE:	SET 1		SET 2		SET 3		SET 4	
	REPS	WEIGHT	REPS	WEIGHT	REPS	WEIGHT	REPS	WEIGHT

CARDIO:	TIME	DISTANCE	PACE	HR

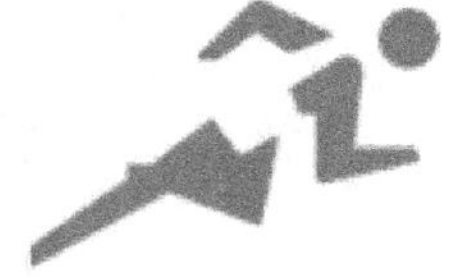

NAME:

DATE:

TIME START:

TIME END:

WARM-UP	TIME	NOTES

STRETCH:	TIME	NOTES

EXERCISE:	SET 1		SET 2		SET 3		SET 4	
	REPS	WEIGHT	REPS	WEIGHT	REPS	WEIGHT	REPS	WEIGHT

CARDIO:	TIME	DISTANCE	PACE	HR

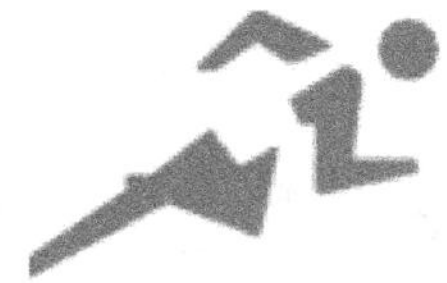

NAME:

DATE:

TIME START:

TIME END:

WARM-UP	TIME	NOTES

STRETCH:	TIME	NOTES

EXERCISE:	SET 1		SET 2		SET 3		SET 4	
	REPS	WEIGHT	REPS	WEIGHT	REPS	WEIGHT	REPS	WEIGHT

CARDIO:	TIME	DISTANCE	PACE	HR

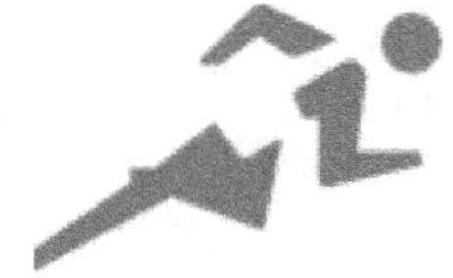

NAME:

DATE:

TIME START:

TIME END:

WARM-UP	TIME	NOTES

STRETCH:	TIME	NOTES

EXERCISE:	SET 1		SET 2		SET 3		SET 4	
	REPS	WEIGHT	REPS	WEIGHT	REPS	WEIGHT	REPS	WEIGHT

CARDIO:	TIME	DISTANCE	PACE	HR

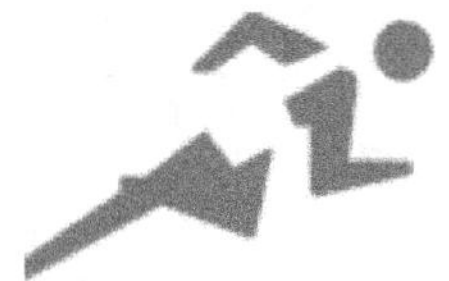

NAME:

DATE:

TIME START:

TIME END:

WARM-UP	TIME	NOTES

STRETCH:	TIME	NOTES

EXERCISE:	SET 1		SET 2		SET 3		SET 4	
	REPS	WEIGHT	REPS	WEIGHT	REPS	WEIGHT	REPS	WEIGHT

CARDIO:	TIME	DISTANCE	PACE	HR

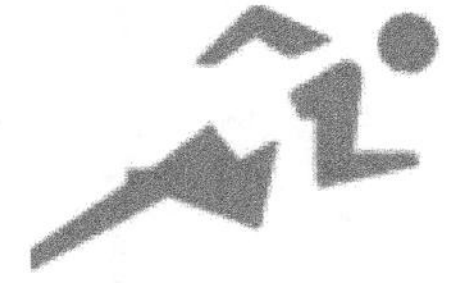

NAME:

DATE:

TIME START:

TIME END:

WARM-UP	TIME	NOTES

STRETCH:	TIME	NOTES

EXERCISE:	SET 1		SET 2		SET 3		SET 4	
	REPS	WEIGHT	REPS	WEIGHT	REPS	WEIGHT	REPS	WEIGHT

CARDIO:	TIME	DISTANCE	PACE	HR

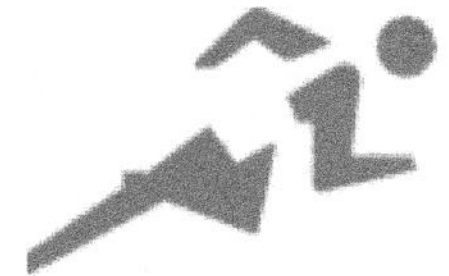

NAME:

DATE:

TIME START:

TIME END:

WARM-UP	TIME	NOTES

STRETCH:	TIME	NOTES

EXERCISE:	SET 1		SET 2		SET 3		SET 4	
	REPS	WEIGHT	REPS	WEIGHT	REPS	WEIGHT	REPS	WEIGHT

CARDIO:	TIME	DISTANCE	PACE	HR

NAME:

DATE:

TIME START:

TIME END:

WARM-UP	TIME	NOTES

STRETCH:	TIME	NOTES

EXERCISE:	SET 1		SET 2		SET 3		SET 4	
	REPS	WEIGHT	REPS	WEIGHT	REPS	WEIGHT	REPS	WEIGHT

CARDIO:	TIME	DISTANCE	PACE	HR

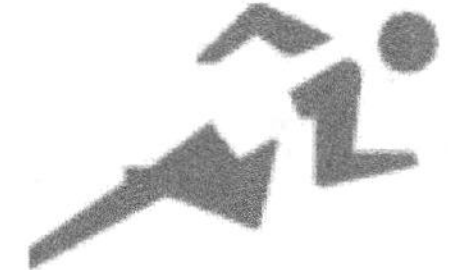

NAME: _______________

DATE: _______________

TIME START: _______________

TIME END: _______________

WARM-UP	TIME	NOTES

STRETCH:	TIME	NOTES

EXERCISE:	SET 1		SET 2		SET 3		SET 4	
	REPS	WEIGHT	REPS	WEIGHT	REPS	WEIGHT	REPS	WEIGHT

CARDIO:	TIME	DISTANCE	PACE	HR

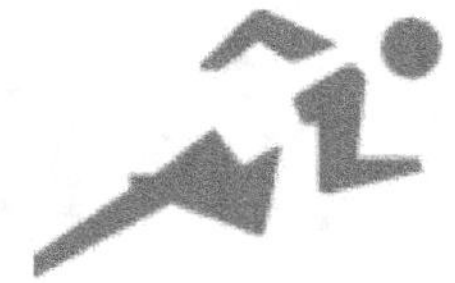

NAME:

DATE:

TIME START:

TIME END:

WARM-UP	TIME	NOTES

STRETCH:	TIME	NOTES

EXERCISE:	SET 1		SET 2		SET 3		SET 4	
	REPS	WEIGHT	REPS	WEIGHT	REPS	WEIGHT	REPS	WEIGHT

CARDIO:	TIME	DISTANCE	PACE	HR

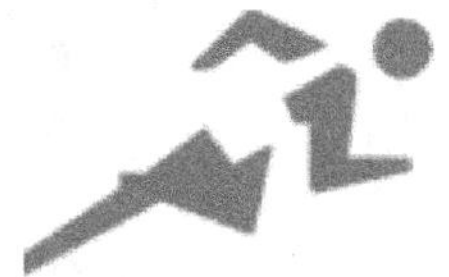

NAME:

DATE:

TIME START:

TIME END:

WARM-UP	TIME	NOTES

STRETCH:	TIME	NOTES

EXERCISE:	SET 1		SET 2		SET 3		SET 4	
	REPS	WEIGHT	REPS	WEIGHT	REPS	WEIGHT	REPS	WEIGHT

CARDIO:	TIME	DISTANCE	PACE	HR

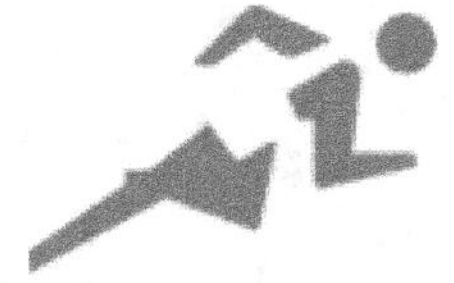

NAME: _______________

DATE: _______________

TIME START: _______________

TIME END: _______________

WARM-UP	TIME	NOTES

STRETCH:	TIME	NOTES

EXERCISE:	SET 1		SET 2		SET 3		SET 4	
	REPS	WEIGHT	REPS	WEIGHT	REPS	WEIGHT	REPS	WEIGHT

CARDIO:	TIME	DISTANCE	PACE	HR

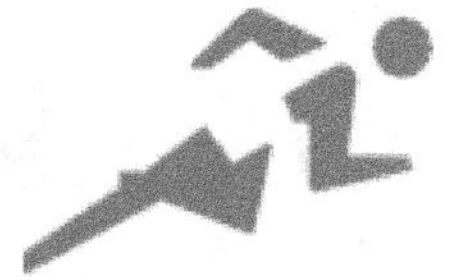

NAME:

DATE:

TIME START:

TIME END:

WARM-UP	TIME	NOTES

STRETCH:	TIME	NOTES

EXERCISE:	SET 1		SET 2		SET 3		SET 4	
	REPS	WEIGHT	REPS	WEIGHT	REPS	WEIGHT	REPS	WEIGHT

CARDIO:	TIME	DISTANCE	PACE	HR

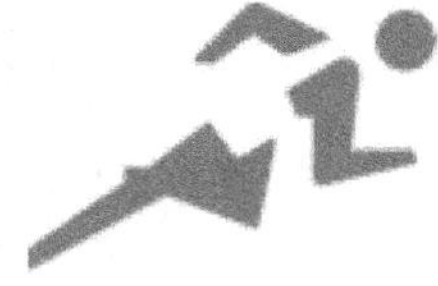

NAME:

DATE:

TIME START:

TIME END:

WARM-UP	TIME	NOTES

STRETCH:	TIME	NOTES

EXERCISE:	SET 1		SET 2		SET 3		SET 4	
	REPS	WEIGHT	REPS	WEIGHT	REPS	WEIGHT	REPS	WEIGHT

CARDIO:	TIME	DISTANCE	PACE	HR

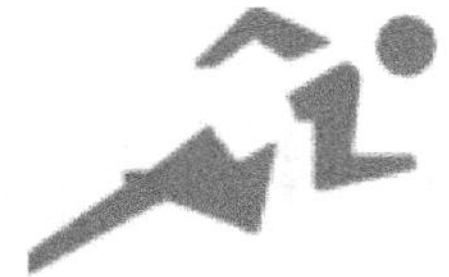

NAME:

DATE:

TIME START:

TIME END:

WARM-UP	TIME	NOTES

STRETCH:	TIME	NOTES

EXERCISE:	SET 1		SET 2		SET 3		SET 4	
	REPS	WEIGHT	REPS	WEIGHT	REPS	WEIGHT	REPS	WEIGHT

CARDIO:	TIME	DISTANCE	PACE	HR

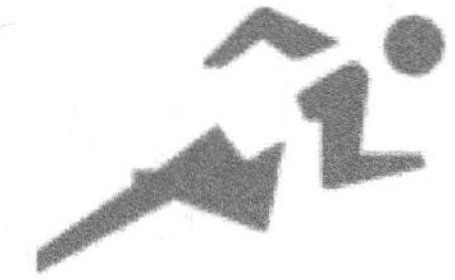

NAME:

DATE:

TIME START:

TIME END:

WARM-UP	TIME	NOTES

STRETCH:	TIME	NOTES

EXERCISE:	SET 1		SET 2		SET 3		SET 4	
	REPS	WEIGHT	REPS	WEIGHT	REPS	WEIGHT	REPS	WEIGHT

CARDIO:	TIME	DISTANCE	PACE	HR

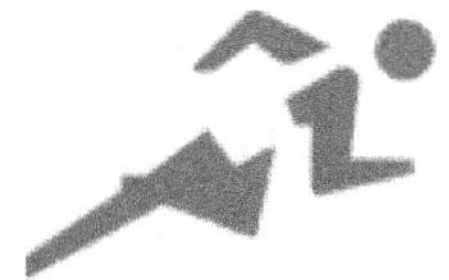

NAME:
DATE:
TIME START:
TIME END:

WARM-UP	TIME	NOTES

STRETCH:	TIME	NOTES

EXERCISE:	SET 1		SET 2		SET 3		SET 4	
	REPS	WEIGHT	REPS	WEIGHT	REPS	WEIGHT	REPS	WEIGHT

CARDIO:	TIME	DISTANCE	PACE	HR

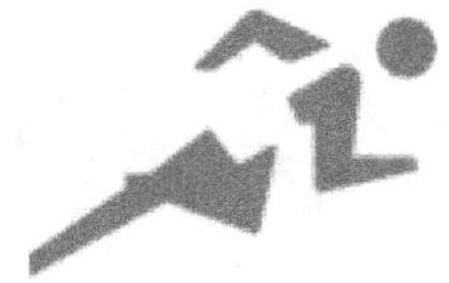

NAME:

DATE:

TIME START:

TIME END:

WARM-UP	TIME	NOTES

STRETCH:	TIME	NOTES

EXERCISE:	SET 1		SET 2		SET 3		SET 4	
	REPS	WEIGHT	REPS	WEIGHT	REPS	WEIGHT	REPS	WEIGHT

CARDIO:	TIME	DISTANCE	PACE	HR

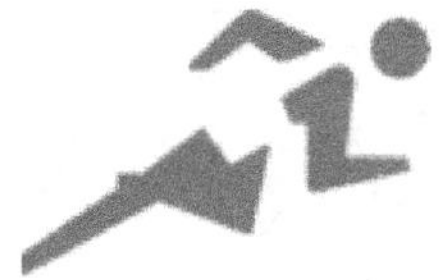

NAME:

DATE:

TIME START:

TIME END:

WARM-UP	TIME	NOTES

STRETCH:	TIME	NOTES

EXERCISE:	SET 1		SET 2		SET 3		SET 4	
	REPS	WEIGHT	REPS	WEIGHT	REPS	WEIGHT	REPS	WEIGHT

CARDIO:	TIME	DISTANCE	PACE	HR

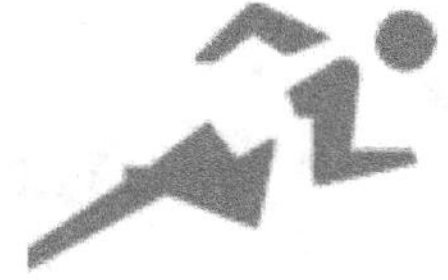

NAME:

DATE:

TIME START:

TIME END:

WARM-UP	TIME	NOTES

STRETCH:	TIME	NOTES

EXERCISE:	SET 1		SET 2		SET 3		SET 4	
	REPS	WEIGHT	REPS	WEIGHT	REPS	WEIGHT	REPS	WEIGHT

CARDIO:	TIME	DISTANCE	PACE	HR

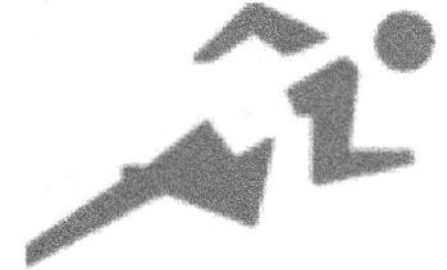

NAME:

DATE:

TIME START:

TIME END:

WARM-UP	TIME	NOTES

STRETCH:	TIME	NOTES

EXERCISE:	SET 1		SET 2		SET 3		SET 4	
	REPS	WEIGHT	REPS	WEIGHT	REPS	WEIGHT	REPS	WEIGHT

CARDIO:	TIME	DISTANCE	PACE	HR

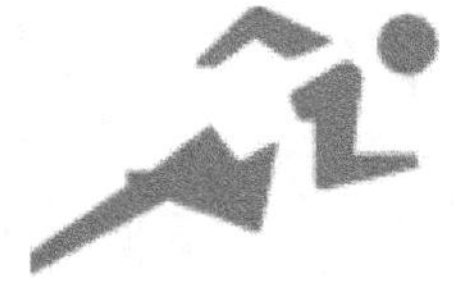

WARM-UP	TIME	NOTES

STRETCH:	TIME	NOTES

EXERCISE:	SET 1		SET 2		SET 3		SET 4	
	REPS	WEIGHT	REPS	WEIGHT	REPS	WEIGHT	REPS	WEIGHT

CARDIO:	TIME	DISTANCE	PACE	HR

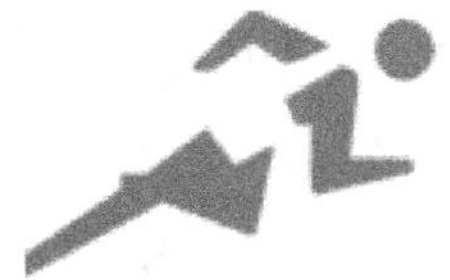

NAME:

DATE:

TIME START:

TIME END:

WARM-UP	TIME	NOTES

STRETCH:	TIME	NOTES

EXERCISE:	SET 1		SET 2		SET 3		SET 4	
	REPS	WEIGHT	REPS	WEIGHT	REPS	WEIGHT	REPS	WEIGHT

CARDIO:	TIME	DISTANCE	PACE	HR

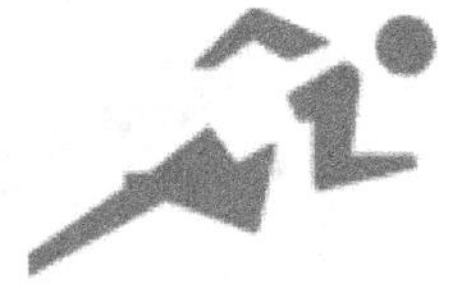

NAME:

DATE:

TIME START:

TIME END:

WARM-UP	TIME	NOTES

STRETCH:	TIME	NOTES

EXERCISE:	SET 1		SET 2		SET 3		SET 4	
	REPS	WEIGHT	REPS	WEIGHT	REPS	WEIGHT	REPS	WEIGHT

CARDIO:	TIME	DISTANCE	PACE	HR

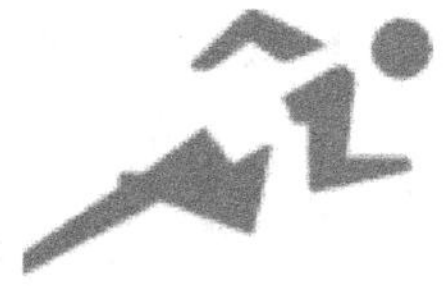

NAME:

DATE:

TIME START:

TIME END:

WARM-UP	TIME	NOTES

STRETCH:	TIME	NOTES

EXERCISE:	SET 1		SET 2		SET 3		SET 4	
	REPS	WEIGHT	REPS	WEIGHT	REPS	WEIGHT	REPS	WEIGHT

CARDIO:	TIME	DISTANCE	PACE	HR

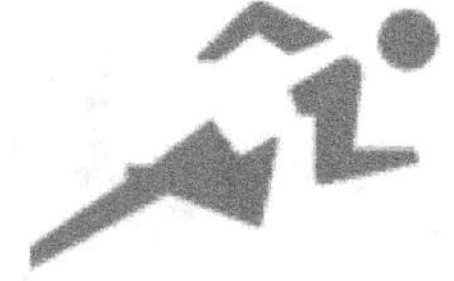

NAME:

DATE:

TIME START:

TIME END:

WARM-UP	TIME	NOTES

STRETCH:	TIME	NOTES

EXERCISE:	SET 1		SET 2		SET 3		SET 4	
	REPS	WEIGHT	REPS	WEIGHT	REPS	WEIGHT	REPS	WEIGHT

CARDIO:	TIME	DISTANCE	PACE	HR

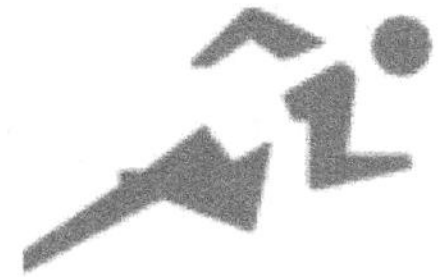

NAME:

DATE:

TIME START:

TIME END:

WARM-UP	TIME	NOTES

STRETCH:	TIME	NOTES

EXERCISE:	SET 1		SET 2		SET 3		SET 4	
	REPS	WEIGHT	REPS	WEIGHT	REPS	WEIGHT	REPS	WEIGHT

CARDIO:	TIME	DISTANCE	PACE	HR

NAME:

DATE:

TIME START:

TIME END:

WARM-UP	TIME	NOTES

STRETCH:	TIME	NOTES

EXERCISE:	SET 1		SET 2		SET 3		SET 4	
	REPS	WEIGHT	REPS	WEIGHT	REPS	WEIGHT	REPS	WEIGHT

CARDIO:	TIME	DISTANCE	PACE	HR

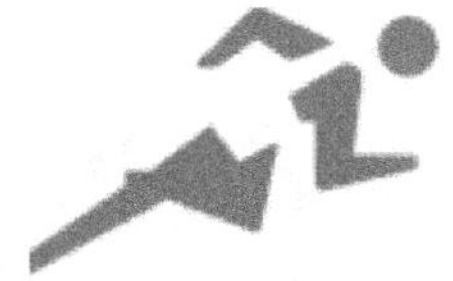

NAME:

DATE:

TIME START:

TIME END:

WARM-UP	TIME	NOTES

STRETCH:	TIME	NOTES

EXERCISE:	SET 1		SET 2		SET 3		SET 4	
	REPS	WEIGHT	REPS	WEIGHT	REPS	WEIGHT	REPS	WEIGHT

CARDIO:	TIME	DISTANCE	PACE	HR

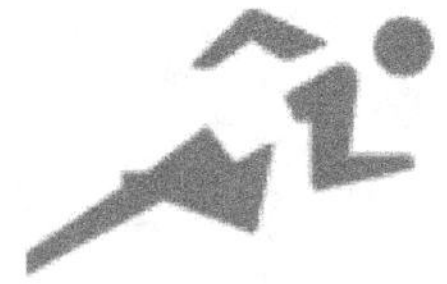

NAME:

DATE:

TIME START:

TIME END:

WARM-UP	TIME	NOTES

STRETCH:	TIME	NOTES

EXERCISE:	SET 1		SET 2		SET 3		SET 4	
	REPS	WEIGHT	REPS	WEIGHT	REPS	WEIGHT	REPS	WEIGHT

CARDIO:	TIME	DISTANCE	PACE	HR

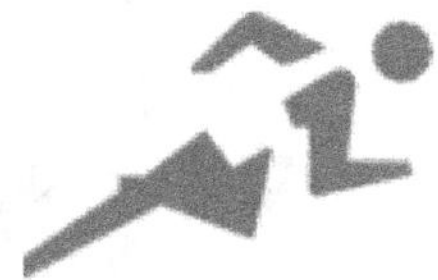

NAME:
DATE:
TIME START:
TIME END:

WARM-UP	TIME	NOTES

STRETCH:	TIME	NOTES

EXERCISE:	SET 1		SET 2		SET 3		SET 4	
	REPS	WEIGHT	REPS	WEIGHT	REPS	WEIGHT	REPS	WEIGHT

CARDIO:	TIME	DISTANCE	PACE	HR

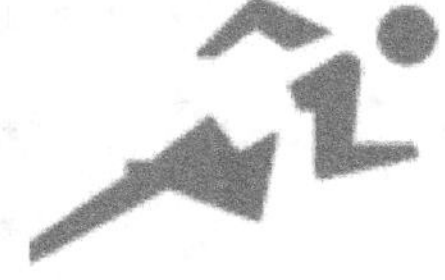

NAME:

DATE:

TIME START:

TIME END:

WARM-UP	TIME	NOTES

STRETCH:	TIME	NOTES

EXERCISE:	SET 1		SET 2		SET 3		SET 4	
	REPS	WEIGHT	REPS	WEIGHT	REPS	WEIGHT	REPS	WEIGHT

CARDIO:	TIME	DISTANCE	PACE	HR

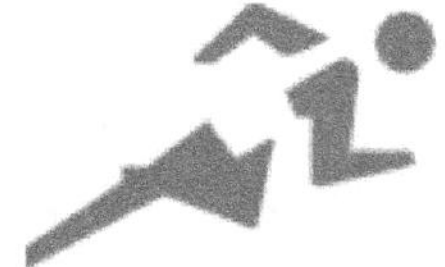

NAME: ______________

DATE: ______________

TIME START: ______________

TIME END: ______________

WARM-UP	TIME	NOTES

STRETCH:	TIME	NOTES

EXERCISE:	SET 1		SET 2		SET 3		SET 4	
	REPS	WEIGHT	REPS	WEIGHT	REPS	WEIGHT	REPS	WEIGHT

CARDIO:	TIME	DISTANCE	PACE	HR

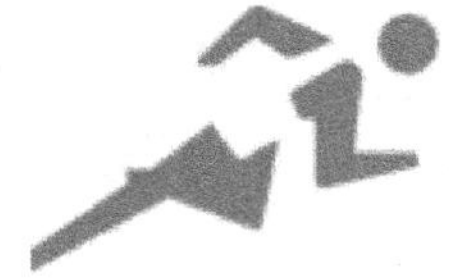

NAME:

DATE:

TIME START:

TIME END:

WARM-UP	TIME	NOTES

STRETCH:	TIME	NOTES

EXERCISE:	SET 1		SET 2		SET 3		SET 4	
	REPS	WEIGHT	REPS	WEIGHT	REPS	WEIGHT	REPS	WEIGHT

CARDIO:	TIME	DISTANCE	PACE	HR

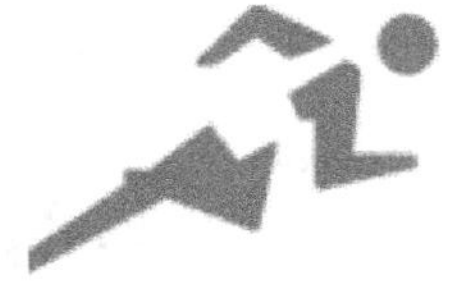

NAME:

DATE:

TIME START:

TIME END:

WARM-UP	TIME	NOTES

STRETCH:	TIME	NOTES

EXERCISE:	SET 1		SET 2		SET 3		SET 4	
	REPS	WEIGHT	REPS	WEIGHT	REPS	WEIGHT	REPS	WEIGHT

CARDIO:	TIME	DISTANCE	PACE	HR

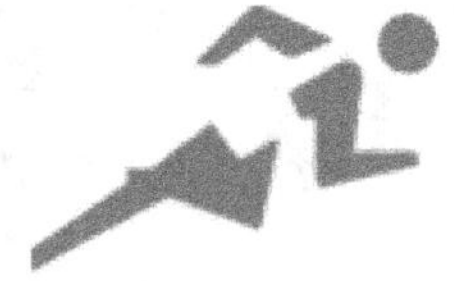

NAME:

DATE:

TIME START:

TIME END:

WARM-UP	TIME	NOTES

STRETCH:	TIME	NOTES

EXERCISE:	SET 1		SET 2		SET 3		SET 4	
	REPS	WEIGHT	REPS	WEIGHT	REPS	WEIGHT	REPS	WEIGHT

CARDIO:	TIME	DISTANCE	PACE	HR

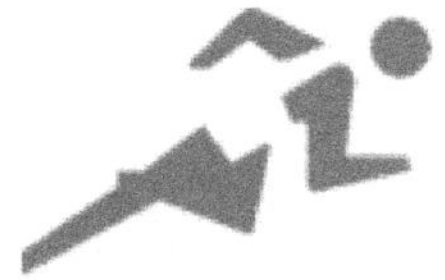

NAME:

DATE:

TIME START:

TIME END:

WARM-UP	TIME	NOTES

STRETCH:	TIME	NOTES

EXERCISE:	SET 1		SET 2		SET 3		SET 4	
	REPS	WEIGHT	REPS	WEIGHT	REPS	WEIGHT	REPS	WEIGHT

CARDIO:	TIME	DISTANCE	PACE	HR

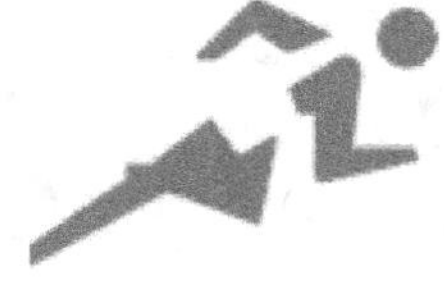

NAME:

DATE:

TIME START:

TIME END:

WARM-UP	TIME	NOTES

STRETCH:	TIME	NOTES

EXERCISE:	SET 1		SET 2		SET 3		SET 4	
	REPS	WEIGHT	REPS	WEIGHT	REPS	WEIGHT	REPS	WEIGHT

CARDIO:	TIME	DISTANCE	PACE	HR

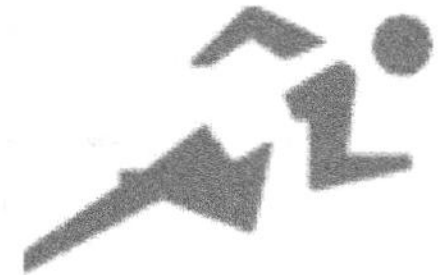

NAME: _______________

DATE: _______________

TIME START: _______________

TIME END: _______________

WARM-UP	TIME	NOTES

STRETCH:	TIME	NOTES

EXERCISE:	SET 1		SET 2		SET 3		SET 4	
	REPS	WEIGHT	REPS	WEIGHT	REPS	WEIGHT	REPS	WEIGHT

CARDIO:	TIME	DISTANCE	PACE	HR

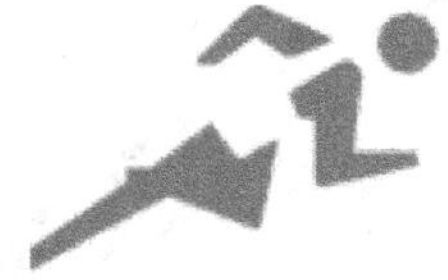

NAME:

DATE:

TIME START:

TIME END:

WARM-UP	TIME	NOTES

STRETCH:	TIME	NOTES

EXERCISE:	SET 1		SET 2		SET 3		SET 4	
	REPS	WEIGHT	REPS	WEIGHT	REPS	WEIGHT	REPS	WEIGHT

CARDIO:	TIME	DISTANCE	PACE	HR

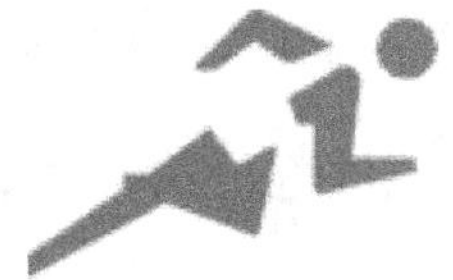

NAME:

DATE:

TIME START:

TIME END:

WARM-UP	TIME	NOTES

STRETCH:	TIME	NOTES

EXERCISE:	SET 1		SET 2		SET 3		SET 4	
	REPS	WEIGHT	REPS	WEIGHT	REPS	WEIGHT	REPS	WEIGHT

CARDIO:	TIME	DISTANCE	PACE	HR

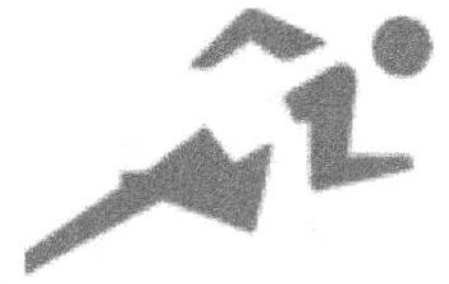

NAME:

DATE:

TIME START:

TIME END:

WARM-UP	TIME	NOTES

STRETCH:	TIME	NOTES

EXERCISE:	SET 1		SET 2		SET 3		SET 4	
	REPS	WEIGHT	REPS	WEIGHT	REPS	WEIGHT	REPS	WEIGHT

CARDIO:	TIME	DISTANCE	PACE	HR

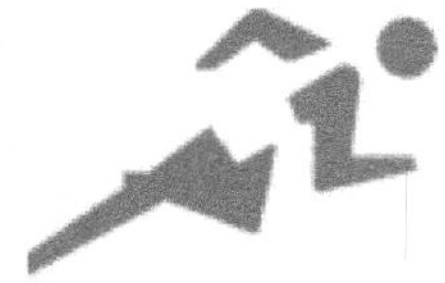

NAME:

DATE:

TIME START:

TIME END:

WARM-UP	TIME	NOTES

STRETCH:	TIME	NOTES

EXERCISE:	SET 1		SET 2		SET 3		SET 4	
	REPS	WEIGHT	REPS	WEIGHT	REPS	WEIGHT	REPS	WEIGHT

CARDIO:	TIME	DISTANCE	PACE	HR

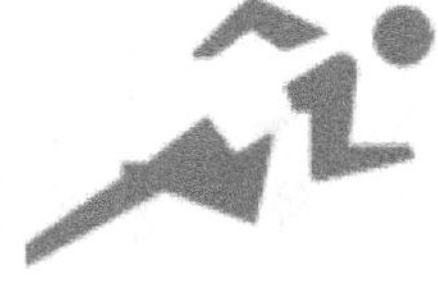

NAME:

DATE:

TIME START:

TIME END:

WARM-UP	TIME	NOTES

STRETCH:	TIME	NOTES

EXERCISE:	SET 1		SET 2		SET 3		SET 4	
	REPS	WEIGHT	REPS	WEIGHT	REPS	WEIGHT	REPS	WEIGHT

CARDIO:	TIME	DISTANCE	PACE	HR

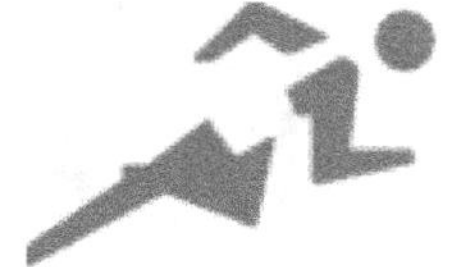

NAME:

DATE:

TIME START:

TIME END:

WARM-UP	TIME	NOTES

STRETCH:	TIME	NOTES

EXERCISE:	SET 1		SET 2		SET 3		SET 4	
	REPS	WEIGHT	REPS	WEIGHT	REPS	WEIGHT	REPS	WEIGHT

CARDIO:	TIME	DISTANCE	PACE	HR

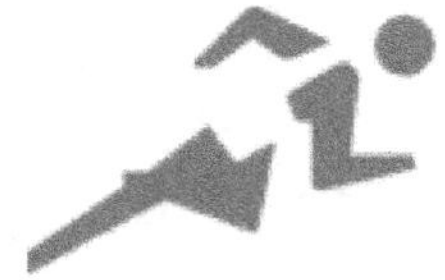

NAME:_______________________

DATE:_______________________

TIME START:_______________________

TIME END:_______________________

WARM-UP	TIME	NOTES

STRETCH:	TIME	NOTES

EXERCISE:	SET 1		SET 2		SET 3		SET 4	
	REPS	WEIGHT	REPS	WEIGHT	REPS	WEIGHT	REPS	WEIGHT

CARDIO:	TIME	DISTANCE	PACE	HR

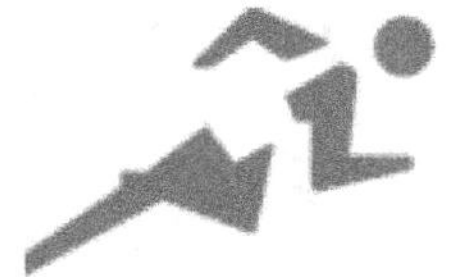

NAME: ___________________

DATE: ___________________

TIME START: ___________________

TIME END: ___________________

WARM-UP	TIME	NOTES

STRETCH:	TIME	NOTES

EXERCISE:	SET 1		SET 2		SET 3		SET 4	
	REPS	WEIGHT	REPS	WEIGHT	REPS	WEIGHT	REPS	WEIGHT

CARDIO:	TIME	DISTANCE	PACE	HR

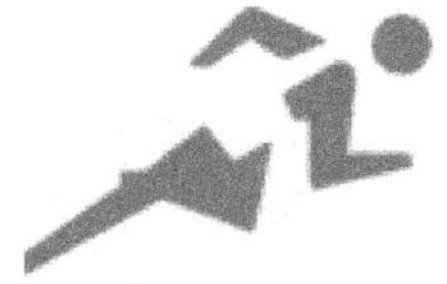

NAME:

DATE:

TIME START:

TIME END:

WARM-UP	TIME	NOTES

STRETCH:	TIME	NOTES

EXERCISE:	SET 1		SET 2		SET 3		SET 4	
	REPS	WEIGHT	REPS	WEIGHT	REPS	WEIGHT	REPS	WEIGHT

CARDIO:	TIME	DISTANCE	PACE	HR

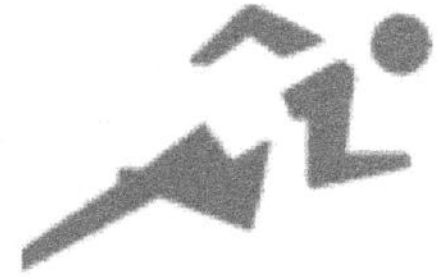

NAME:

DATE:

TIME START:

TIME END:

WARM-UP	TIME	NOTES

STRETCH:	TIME	NOTES

EXERCISE:	SET 1		SET 2		SET 3		SET 4	
	REPS	WEIGHT	REPS	WEIGHT	REPS	WEIGHT	REPS	WEIGHT

CARDIO:	TIME	DISTANCE	PACE	HR

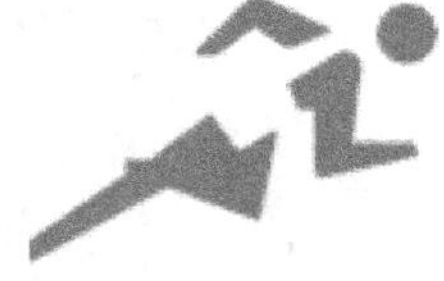

NAME:

DATE:

TIME START:

TIME END:

WARM-UP	TIME	NOTES

STRETCH:	TIME	NOTES

EXERCISE:	SET 1		SET 2		SET 3		SET 4	
	REPS	WEIGHT	REPS	WEIGHT	REPS	WEIGHT	REPS	WEIGHT

CARDIO:	TIME	DISTANCE	PACE	HR

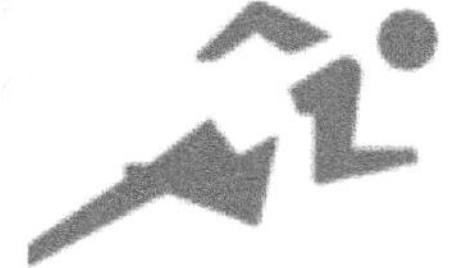

NAME:
DATE:
TIME START:
TIME END:

WARM-UP	TIME	NOTES

STRETCH:	TIME	NOTES

EXERCISE:	SET 1		SET 2		SET 3		SET 4	
	REPS	WEIGHT	REPS	WEIGHT	REPS	WEIGHT	REPS	WEIGHT

CARDIO:	TIME	DISTANCE	PACE	HR

NAME:

DATE:

TIME START:

TIME END:

WARM-UP	TIME	NOTES

STRETCH:	TIME	NOTES

EXERCISE:	SET 1		SET 2		SET 3		SET 4	
	REPS	WEIGHT	REPS	WEIGHT	REPS	WEIGHT	REPS	WEIGHT

CARDIO:	TIME	DISTANCE	PACE	HR

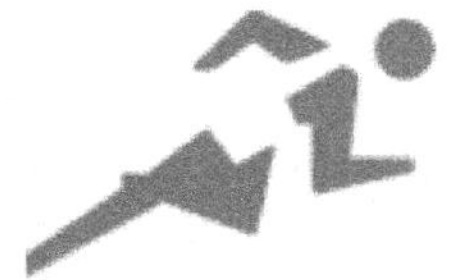

NAME:

DATE:

TIME START:

TIME END:

WARM-UP	TIME	NOTES

STRETCH:	TIME	NOTES

EXERCISE:	SET 1		SET 2		SET 3		SET 4	
	REPS	WEIGHT	REPS	WEIGHT	REPS	WEIGHT	REPS	WEIGHT

CARDIO:	TIME	DISTANCE	PACE	HR

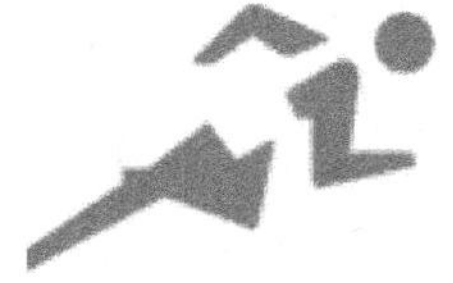

NAME:

DATE:

TIME START:

TIME END:

WARM-UP	TIME	NOTES

STRETCH:	TIME	NOTES

EXERCISE:	SET 1		SET 2		SET 3		SET 4	
	REPS	WEIGHT	REPS	WEIGHT	REPS	WEIGHT	REPS	WEIGHT

CARDIO:	TIME	DISTANCE	PACE	HR

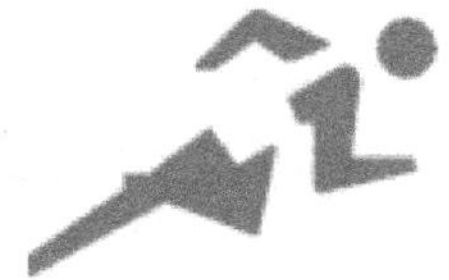

NAME:

DATE:

TIME START:

TIME END:

WARM-UP	TIME	NOTES

STRETCH:	TIME	NOTES

EXERCISE:	SET 1		SET 2		SET 3		SET 4	
	REPS	WEIGHT	REPS	WEIGHT	REPS	WEIGHT	REPS	WEIGHT

CARDIO:	TIME	DISTANCE	PACE	HR

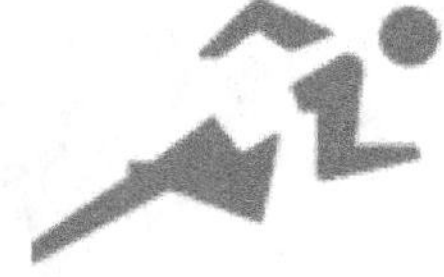

NAME:

DATE:

TIME START:

TIME END:

WARM-UP	TIME	NOTES

STRETCH:	TIME	NOTES

EXERCISE:	SET 1		SET 2		SET 3		SET 4	
	REPS	WEIGHT	REPS	WEIGHT	REPS	WEIGHT	REPS	WEIGHT

CARDIO:	TIME	DISTANCE	PACE	HR

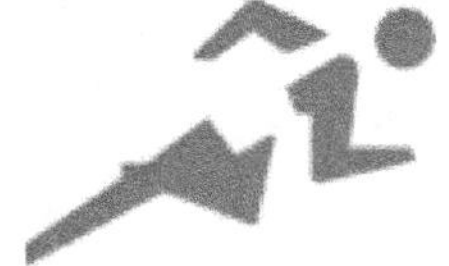

NAME:

DATE:

TIME START:

TIME END:

WARM-UP	TIME	NOTES

STRETCH:	TIME	NOTES

EXERCISE:	SET 1		SET 2		SET 3		SET 4	
	REPS	WEIGHT	REPS	WEIGHT	REPS	WEIGHT	REPS	WEIGHT

CARDIO:	TIME	DISTANCE	PACE	HR

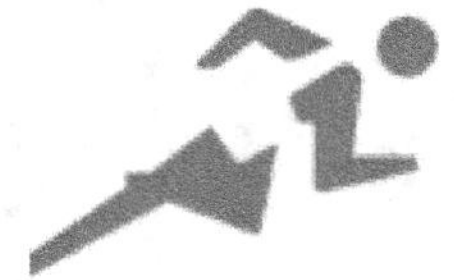

NAME:________________

DATE:________________

TIME START:________________

TIME END:________________

WARM-UP	TIME	NOTES

STRETCH:	TIME	NOTES

EXERCISE:	SET 1		SET 2		SET 3		SET 4	
	REPS	WEIGHT	REPS	WEIGHT	REPS	WEIGHT	REPS	WEIGHT

CARDIO:	TIME	DISTANCE	PACE	HR

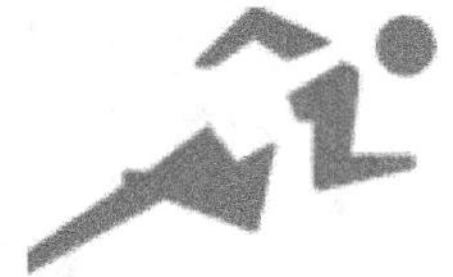

NAME:

DATE:

TIME START:

TIME END:

WARM-UP	TIME	NOTES

STRETCH:	TIME	NOTES

EXERCISE:	SET 1		SET 2		SET 3		SET 4	
	REPS	WEIGHT	REPS	WEIGHT	REPS	WEIGHT	REPS	WEIGHT

CARDIO:	TIME	DISTANCE	PACE	HR

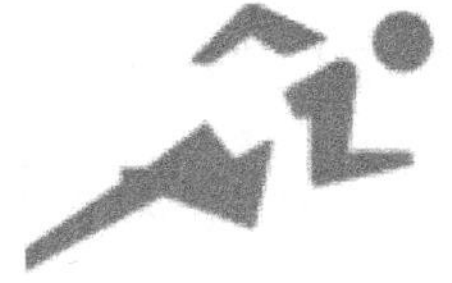

NAME:

DATE:

TIME START:

TIME END:

WARM-UP	TIME	NOTES

STRETCH:	TIME	NOTES

EXERCISE:	SET 1		SET 2		SET 3		SET 4	
	REPS	WEIGHT	REPS	WEIGHT	REPS	WEIGHT	REPS	WEIGHT

CARDIO:	TIME	DISTANCE	PACE	HR

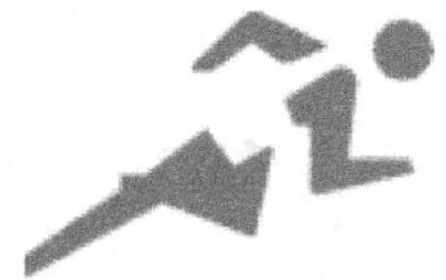

NAME: __________

DATE: __________

TIME START: __________

TIME END: __________

WARM-UP	TIME	NOTES

STRETCH:	TIME	NOTES

EXERCISE:	SET 1		SET 2		SET 3		SET 4	
	REPS	WEIGHT	REPS	WEIGHT	REPS	WEIGHT	REPS	WEIGHT

CARDIO:	TIME	DISTANCE	PACE	HR

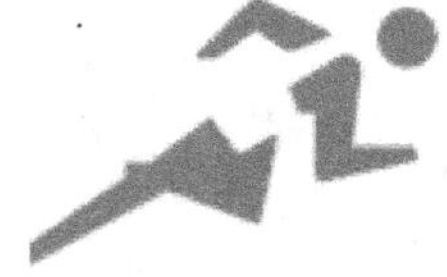

NAME:

DATE:

TIME START:

TIME END:

WARM-UP	TIME	NOTES

STRETCH:	TIME	NOTES

EXERCISE:	SET 1		SET 2		SET 3		SET 4	
	REPS	WEIGHT	REPS	WEIGHT	REPS	WEIGHT	REPS	WEIGHT

CARDIO:	TIME	DISTANCE	PACE	HR